I0791005

Terms and Conditions

Table Of Contents

Foreword

In this EBook I will try to demonstrate different techniques of yoga. Especially if you have never tried it before then, this EBook will be the best thing to start with because I am going to tell you very basic techniques of yoga. If you want to define yoga then, you will come across different definitions by different people.

Some people say that it is reunion of outer winds with the inner body and some say that it is the way of getting inner peace. You will find one thing common in almost every yoga definition that they talk about inner peace and inner self in it. This is basic theme of yoga that you have to become familiar with your inner person.

The basic meaning of yoga is union and you can say that it unites your body, spirit and thoughts. There are so many techniques in this art of exercise and all of these techniques are considered very effective but you should start from basic because if you adopted some advanced technique from start then, it will become difficult for you and you will lose control over it.

All of these yoga exercises make you believe that you exist and you exist with lots of strength and courage. It allows you to gather all of that strength and courage and accomplish your goal in your life.

People who practice personal productivity also utilize yoga as a very effective technique to increase their focus. If you feel tiredness too often or you feel fatigue after a tiring day at office then, you must practice yoga and you will see a new change in yourself and your working ability will also be boosted.

Yoga originated from India and its surrounding regions but then, it spread throughout the world because it has a strong connection with spirituality and everyone wants to get closer to their inner self.

Getting to know you is difficult and especially in today's artificial and superficial world, it is really difficult to live with yourself. You always have to go through family pressures and social pressures and you are forced to do things which you often do not like. Yoga allows you to ease all of those pressures and be very light internally.

Yoga For Beginners

Baby Steps For Practicing And Discovering The Joy Of Yoga

Chapter 1:
Introduction to Yoga

Synopsis

You will learn the basic techniques and concepts of yoga in this chapter.

- ☐ Exercise
- ☐ Breathing techniques
- ☐ Meditation techniques

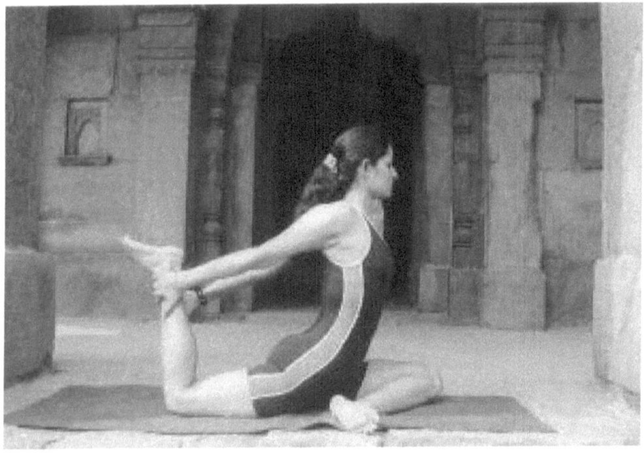

The Basics

Yoga is basically an ancient knowledge of body which originated from Indians and it is more than 500 years old. The basic word of yoga is originated from a Sanskrit word "yuj" which means to unite or to integrate two things. Yoga is exercised and practiced to unite your body with your spirit or you can make it easier and say that the reunion of person's own consciousness and universal consciousness is achieved through yoga.

Ancient people, who practiced yoga, believed in the fact that in order to achieve internal peace, a person must integrate and unite his mind, body and spirit. Without this reunion, person can never achieve internal peace.

This is very dense and difficult process to unite all three of the above because you need extraordinary control over your emotions, intelligence and actions. Yugis developed some easy and short cut ways to achieve balance between intelligence, emotions and actions and this balance was dependent upon three basic things that were exercise, breathing and meditation. These three things are thought to be the pillars of yoga.

Exercise

Human body is treated with lots of respect and care in yoga and this allows the yoga exercises to be very friendly and calming for body structure. Once you start practicing these exercises, then, you will see that there is no twist in these exercises and they are very basic poses which are formulated by yogis to develop peace within the body structure.

Breathing Techniques

Breathing techniques were included in this process because breathing is the source of life and when your source of life is out of order then, how can you expect to have harmony and order in your life.

Breathing techniques help person to gain control over his whole body and his whole internal system as well. These techniques are little difficult to learn but yoga is all about practice and you can learn them by regular practice easily.

Meditation Techniques

Meditation is another thing which is necessary for yoga practice but there is some misconception involved about this technique and people think that their mind has to go blank for meditation.

This is not the case because meditation is just another self-controlling technique which allows you to think more clearly and it harmonizes your thoughts and actions. All three of the above things are very necessary part of yoga and you have to learn all three of the above step by step. You can say these techniques are the stairs to master yoga.

Most of the people become hesitant and say that they have never done any stretching exercise and they cannot learn the difficult poses of yoga but this is a wrong thinking. Yoga is for everyone who wants peace and harmony in his life. There is nothing in this world which is made and designed for specific people instead all humans have equal capabilities and everyone can practice and master yoga.

You just need to concentrate very hard on these skills and integrate them in your life in such a way that they become your habit. There is a saying that you should make yoga so much important part of your life that you may forget to eat but you should never forget to practice yoga.

This saying can tell y9ou the importance of regularity in yoga. The first thing which yoga will give you will be a great looking and perfectly healthy body which everyone wants and after that later stages of breathing techniques and meditation appear.

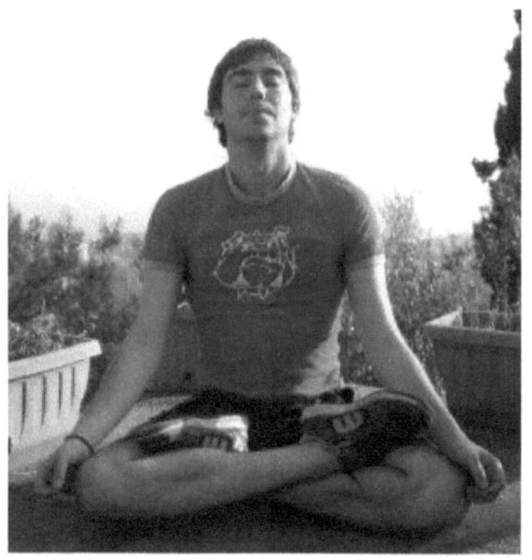

Chapter 2:
Branches of Yoga

Synopsis

There are total six branches of yoga which you can adopt and in this chapter, I will tell you about all of those 6 branches in detail.

- Hatha yoga
- Bhakti yoga
- Raja yoga
- Jnana yoga or yoga of mind
- Karma yoga
- Tantra yoga

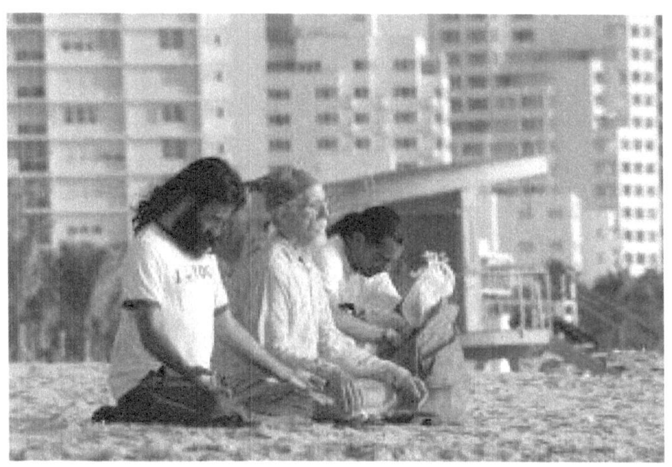

The Kinds

As I mentioned above that Yoga was originated from Indians and it is a very ancient art with lots of skills and complexities involved. If you think that yoga is just about posing your body in difficult positions then, you are mistaken because there are different branches of yoga which are listed below.

Hatha Yoga

Hatha yoga is also called yoga of postures and it is most famous branch of yoga in west which you must have seen. In this branch, body is twisted in different difficult and easy postures. The basic emphasis of this branch is to achieve peace through physical exercises, breathing techniques and mediation. Basic purpose of this yoga branch is to achieve better health along with spirituality.

This is the easiest branch as well because it does not take too much time from your busy routine and you can learn and master this art along with your daily work. You can easily adjust your schedule to practice and your daily routine will not be disturbed with this yoga branch.

Bhakti Yoga

Bhakti yoga is not very popular in the west but it is most practiced branch of yoga in India. This involved spirituality more than physical gestures and it revolves around heart and divine. You have to choose a path which suits your hear desires most and then, you have to see everything and everyone through that path. Bhakti yoga allows you to develop your faith in something and they take that faith to that level where it can tell you the exact way to catch.

Raja Yoga

Raja yoga is also called yoga of self-control. Even though self-control is characteristic of almost every yoga branch but this branch pays special attention to self-control. Most of the people who practice this branch of yoga are members of some religious prestige. Raja yogi sees him as central and gives respect to everything around.

The basic step in mastering self-control is to allow you to be discovered. Discipline learning is the basic characteristic of raja yoga and if your life is distracted and undisciplined then, you must practice raja yoga to gain control of your life and make it more disciplined.

Jnana Yoga or Yoga Of Mind

Jnana yoga which is also called yoga of mind deals primarily with human brain and it tends to control the intelligence of people. In this yoga people learn to integrate wisdom and intellect and with combination of these two, they try to create a perfect moment in their life when they never make wrong decisions. People who practice jnana yoga are very open minded and they keep learning about other religions, professionals, in order to expand their knowledge as they believe that expanding the knowledge expands their mental and intellect strength.

Karma Yoga

Karma yoga believes that you can make your future better by doing kind and selfless deeds in the present. It also believes that if your present is uncertain and hard then, it is the result of your past deeds.

Yogis, who practice karma yoga, do selfless help of other people, in order to make sure that their kindness to other people will make their future a better place. Karma yoga changes their whole concept of good and evil which changes their internal soul and makes them a better person with a bright destiny.

Tantra Yoga

Tantra yoga is the yoga of rituals but most of the times; it is misunderstood by many people because they rename it as sex yoga. Sex is just another part of this yoga but this is not all about tantra yoga. Yogis who practice tantra yoga possess certain qualities like purity, humility, devotion, dedication to his Guru, cosmic love and some others.

These are all the branches of yoga but there are some misconceptions also there about yoga for example some people say yoga is a religion but it is not. Yoga is just a way to make your life better and integrate peace in your life. It helps you to achieve a better life with more control over your mind, thoughts and actions. Yoga is also taken as just an exercise to keep your body fit which is true to some extent but it is not the whole concept of yoga. Exercise and physical health is just small portion of yoga but the higher aim of yoga is lot more sacred and important.

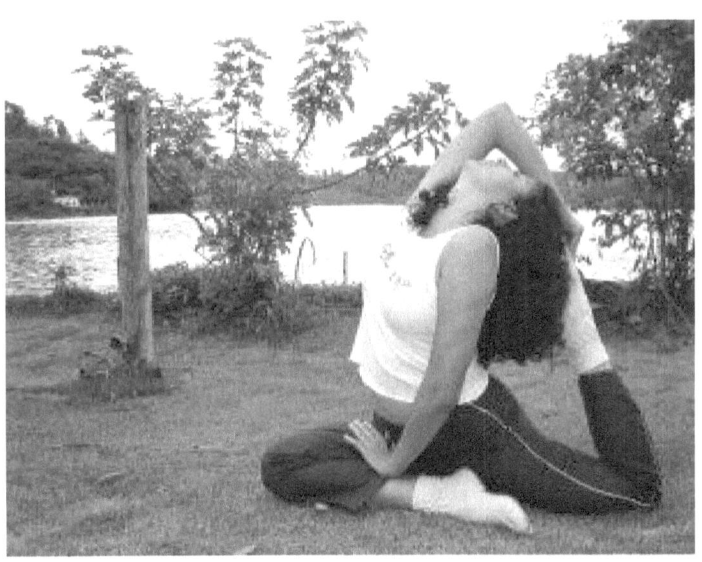

Chapter 3:
Basics of Yoga for Beginners

Synopsis

You will learn some basic stuff and techniques of yoga and if you have never attempted yoga exercises before then, you can start from this.

- Check your physical health status
- Concentrate on just yourself
- Make your mind for physical as well as mental exercises
- Choosing appropriate yoga class
- Commitment is necessary
- Try to find pleasure and fun in yoga classes

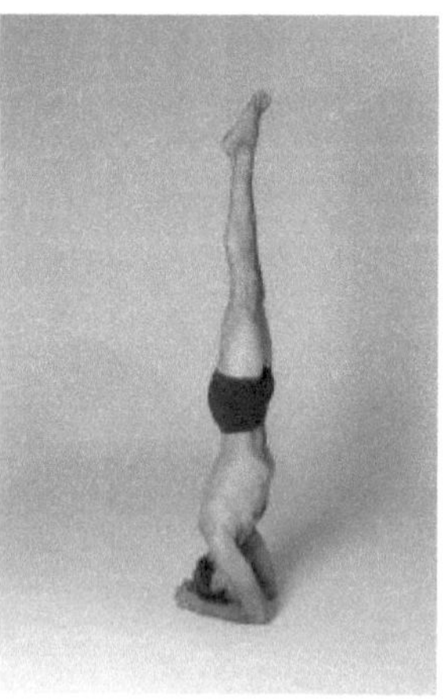

The Beginning

If you are planning to start practice of yoga then, you must know about certain things and in fact if you say more precisely then, there are 6 major things which you must know. These things are listed below and read them carefully for proper implementation of yoga exercises and techniques.

Check Your Physical Health Status

This is basic thing to know about your physical ability. Though the starting work of yoga will not be very tough and anyone can execute it perfectly but as the time passes and you advanced in these techniques, these will keep becoming tougher.

In order to adopt yoga properly, you should have your physical checkup before starting yoga and make sure that you do not execute any techniques which your body does not allow you to do. In this physical checkup, if you find out that you have certain disorder or weakness in some muscle then, you can change your routine accordingly.

Concentrate On Just Yourself

When you join certain yoga learning classes then, you will come across wide range of people and some of them will be way ahead of you in practicing yoga but this should not discourage you from your cause instead, take these classes as personal development area where everyone is responsible for him or herself.

If someone is ahead of you then, this means he or she has practiced more than you and not because he or she is better than you. So concentrate on just yourself and make sure that you are on the right path.

Make Your Mind For Physical As Well As Mental Exercises

Some people have this misconception that yoga is all about physical exercise but this is not entirely true because yoga is about practicing mental exercises as well. You will always have to prepare yourself for that and believe in the fact that yoga is about 50 percent physical and 50 percent mental stamina. It is to create a harmony between your mind and your body. This harmony will need some struggle and hard work to be achieved.

Choosing Appropriate Yoga Class

There are different techniques available for executing in yoga and you need to select one which suits your mood. There are techniques like breathing techniques, mental exercises and even in some cases, laughing is also used to increase strength.

You should do your research about all these techniques and select the one which you think is most interesting for you and you will do it from your heart. Never choose your yoga technique by looking at your friend because he or she may have different interest and this can lead to discouragement.

Commitment is Necessary

Commitment is very necessary in yoga like any other exercise plan because if you keep on changing the technique or you keep missing the classes then, it will disturb the whole schedule and instead of giving you relief and relaxation, this may lead you to unbalanced physical level which can be dangerous. In order to gather most advantage out of yoga, you need to be very consistent about your approach.

Try To Find Pleasure and Fun in Yoga Classes

This is most crucial thing for making your yoga practice very fruitful and effective that you need to enjoy your yoga classes instead of taking them as burden and forcing yourself to go down and practice, you should have a fun attitude and you should wait for these classes to start throughout the day. This approach can change the whole effect of yoga practice and you can see the results by adopting this approach.

Chapter 4:
Poses of Yoga for Beginners

Synopsis

In this chapter, I will demonstrate different poses of yoga which you can practice easily.

- Basics of yoga
- The candles pose
- Mouse pose
- Dog pose
- Cobra pose
- Peacock pose
- Mountain pose
- Butterfly pose
- Birds pose
- Fish pose
- Do nothing doll

Positions

As I mentioned above that hathe yoga which is also called yoga os poses is very famous in the west, so in this chapter, I will tell you some of the basic and also some advanced poses which are exercised in yoga. Before learning these poses, you should learn some safety tips as well because if you exercised these poses in wrong way then, your body will get twisted and you may get hurt as a result.

- You need to be focused while practicing these moves and never think about anything else other that the move.
- Gentle approach should be applied because purpose of these moves is to gain comfort.
- Do not lose concentration and keep practicing.
- Try to observe the poses from pictures and try to perfect your angels.

Basics of Yoga

There are three things which are basic ingredients for learning yoga and these three things are breathing, movement and focus. If you can master and control these three things then, you will be able to learn yoga very fast. Deep breathing is the key and more deeply you breathe, more oxygen you will provide to your muscles and they will be able to adopt the technique. Holding to these difficult poses need a strong body and physical health. You need to be very fit to exercise these poses effectively. You need to make your body very flexible to adopt difficult angels easily. Focus will give you enough power to harmonize both breathing and movement which will create an inner peace for you.

The Candles Pose

In this pose, you have to kneel on your shines and sit on your heels. Pressing your palms and heels together in front of your chest and taking a deep breath is the exact way to do it. You can repeat this pose 3-4 times easily.

Mouse Pose

Kneeling on your shines and sitting back on your heels is start of this pose. Bring chest close to your thighs and let your forehead rest on the floor. Stretch your arms behind you and let them relax. Relax all of your muscles and lay down in same position for some time. This is basically muscle relaxing pose.

Dog Pose

This is an advanced pose which starts from standing on both your arms and legs. Curl your toes and list your hips straight towards ceiling. In this position, you should look like in a V opposition. Your head should be hanging down to observe your own legs. You can learn this by watching a dog stretching after a nap. This pose allows you to strength all of your bones and muscles equally.

Cobra Pose

Lay down on your tummy with your legs straight. Place your arm on either sides and try to lift your chest as high as possible without moving your legs from straight position. Keep the shoulders wide and with an open chest, try to lift it even higher by pressing your hands on the floor. Your head should be straight with the shoulders and this pose can help you to relax your chest muscles as well as shoulders.

Peacock Pose

Sit up tall by widening your legs as wide as possible. Placing hands in front of you and pressing them to widen your shoulders will get you in this pose. This pose is little difficult to adopt but try and hold it for 5 deep breaths.

Mountain Pose

Stand straight up with your feet very close to each other. Bend your neck and look straight up in the ceiling. Let your arms relax on either sides and try to lift your chest. In this position, your head, shoulders and hips should be aligned. This pose is easier and you can hold this pose for 5-10 deep breaths.

Butterfly Pose

Sit by keeping the soles of your feet together. Rest your hands on your shoulders and lift and spread elbows wide. Flap your arms and legs gently like butterfly. You can repeat this process 15-20 times easily.

Birds Pose

In standing position, get your arms behind you and try to lift yourself on toe end of your feet. Be careful because most of the people fall while attempting this posture and you should rise up as much as you can and as soon as you start to lose balance, stop in that position and hold that position for 3-5 deep breaths.

Fish Pose

Lie down on the floor with your legs straight. Place your elbows on either sides and lift your chest with help of elbows as high as you can. Head should be very still and should rest on the floor. This is also a difficult pose and you should hold it for not more than 3 deep breaths.

Do Nothing Doll

Lie on your back in normal position and your arms open and palms facing skies. This is a total relaxing position and normally it is practiced at the end of all poses. Just close your eyes in this pose and try to relax. Think of yourself as a doll which has nothing to move. Stay in this pose for 5-8 minutes in the end of your yoga session.

Chapter 5:
Poses of Yoga for Experts

Synopsis

In above chapter I have described some basic poses which are for beginners and now I am going to teach you some advanced poses which are for pro yogis.

- The bridge yoga pose
- The plough yoga pose
- The forward bend yoga pose
- The locust yoga pose:
- The bow yoga pose
- The half spinal twist yoga pose

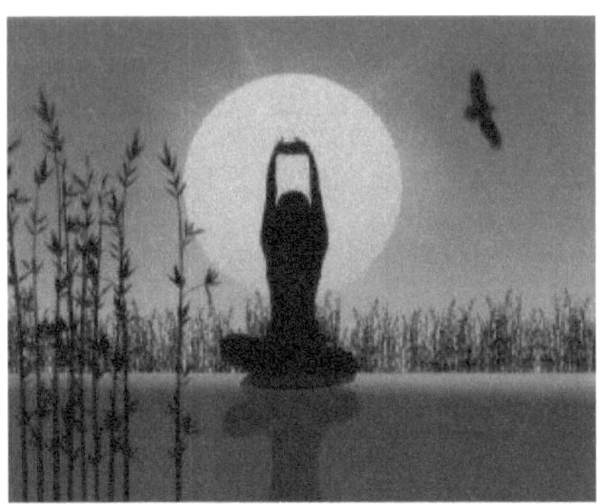

Expert Positions

Once you have progressed from beginner's level to a higher level then, you need to change your poses and exercise some advanced poses because these poses will be more effective on you and you will not feel any trouble in implementing these advanced poses.

The Bridge Yoga Pose

This pose is a difficult pose and it is practiced when you are coming out of shoulder pose. To execute this pose perfectly, you need a very strong spine. If you are weak from your back then, you do not need to execute this pose as it can hurt your back.

The Plough Yoga Pose

This is another advanced pose which is for those people who have developed supreme kind of flexibility and strength in their muscles by practicing all the other ordinary poses of yoga. You can search internet and you will find exact pictures depicting this pose and you can execute it at your own after wards.

The Forward Bend Yoga Pose

This is another very difficult pose and in order to execute it you need to hold the toe ends of your feet for several deep breaths. This is also dangerous for people with any back problems because your back will suffer a full bend and if you have slight problem in your back then, it will invoke that problem.

The Locust Yoga Pose

This is another very tough pose but the difficulty is not in executing it but in holding it for several minutes and as usual, it also needs a very strong back. You should practice on basic poses and develop your back muscles to execute these poses effectively.

The Bow Yoga Pose

This yoga pose is just for expert yogis because it is difficult to execute and even more difficult to hold. You need tons of stamina and back strength which comes from years of practice. If someone challenges you to execute this pose then, you should think twice before accepting the challenge.

The Half Spinal Twist Yoga Pose

As it is evident from the name that it requires your spine to get twisted and to twist your spine, you need a back like rock which should never bother you in any position.

These are some of the yoga poses which are very difficult to execute and if you have noticed something that all of the above mentioned poses require very strong back.

They involve your back in the process somehow which demands that you should practice on regular and easy poses and develop your back so much that you can execute these advanced poses of yoga.

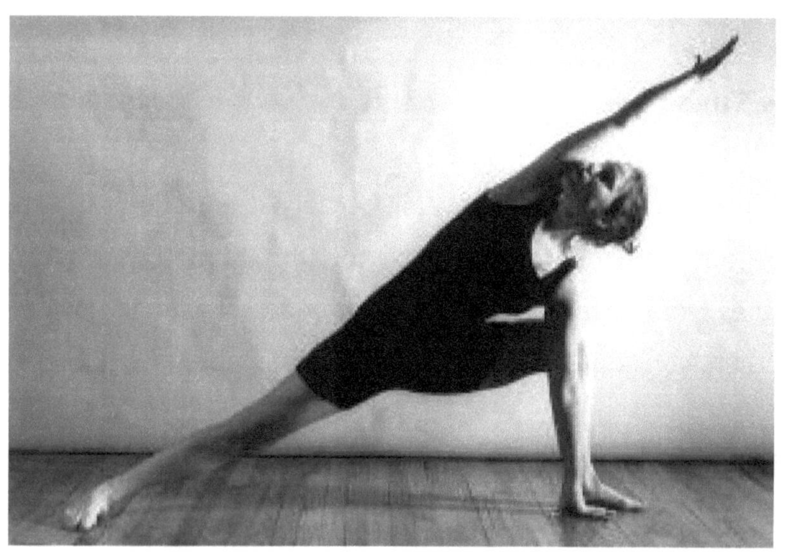

Chapter 6:
An Overview of the Fundamental Principles

Synopsis

In this chapter, I will reveal all the benefits and advantages of yoga which you can get directly or indirectly.

- Increasing flexibility
- Increased use of joints, ligaments and tendons
- Increased strength and weight management
- Improved blood circulation
- Detoxification
- Stress relief and pain relief
- Focus on present and inner peace
- Yoga is beneficial for all age groups
- Better breathing and body awareness

The Precepts

Yoga is taken as a physical remedy for many problems and especially for people, who tend to suffer from different health related problems like pain, stress, fatigue, sleeping disorder and other similar issues, yoga is perfect solution. It just needs a bit of practice and patience to see the results and initially, you can face some problems but as the time passes, you will learn the art of doing exercises properly and will start to relax after doing them. Following are the few advantages which you can get from yoga exercises.

Increasing Flexibility

Getting a flexible body is dream of almost every person but it is very tough to attain certain level of flexibility without proper exercise routine. All the exercises of yoga are based to increase stamina, flexibility and length of your muscles. I have seen people who started yoga when they were not even able to touch their foot toes but after some practice, they were able to bend their back completely without any trouble to touch their toes. Not only this but if you observe different poses of yoga then, you will know that it emphasis on certain parts of body which are almost ignored in daily routine but yoga exercises get these parts activated and makes them flexible to work.

Increased Use of Joints, Ligaments and Tendons

As I mentioned above that yoga increases flexibility and it is because of that long research of yoga positions. Every position is well-thought and well-conceived that you can activate your those parts of the body which are normally ignored for example, shoulder are a part of our body which can change our whole posture but we seldom do any exercise or certain movement which involved shoulders. In yoga, on the other hand, there are special postures which give stress and relax shoulder particularly and ultimately you make your shoulders strong and flexible.

Increased Strength and Weight Management

Yoga exercises help you in increasing the overall strength of all your body parts including your bones. This increased strength increases support for your whole skeleton. This is a great way to achieve a healthy and toned body. It not only increases the overall strength of your body but it also helps you in maintain your weigh because you have to practice different postures every day and in those postures, if your weight increases, you will notice it in very timely manner.

Improved Blood Circulation

Yoga is recommended for patients who have increased blood pressure or even low blood pressure. There are different poses and exercises for both of these purposes. It regulates blood in a more proper way because the positions which are practiced in yoga are very precise and these positions make sure that every organ of the body comes in exact position which makes the job for the heat easier. It circulates the blood more easily and more properly.

Detoxification

In yoga, muscles are stretched very gently and in some techniques massage are done and these techniques ensure proper blood flow in whole body which also works as detoxification of body. All the undesired secretions are effectively removes from the body because everything works in order.

Stress Relief and Pain Relief

Cortisol is a substance in our body which controls the amount of stress and it is seen that all the yoga exercises help to reduce the amount of cortisol in human body which ultimately limits the effects of stress on our body. In ancient times, yoga exercises were used to cure different kinds of pain and in some parts of the world, some expert yogis still practice this technique of lowing and getting rid of pains.

Focus On Present and Inner Peace

Inner peace is a thing which is very rare in this materialistic world and through practice of yoga you can get this rare quality in yourself. Along with physical health, improving mental health is also a future of yoga exercises because it creates a harmony between thoughts, mind and actions of our body. It allows you to converge and focus your thoughts on one purpose of your life. It avoids all the distractions and enables your mind to think very clearly about the success.

Yoga is Beneficial for All Age Groups

If you observe yoga techniques then, you will notice that these techniques are not specific for any age group because some of these are very easy and some of them are complex which shows that people from any age group can practice these techniques and get results. In fact, as you keep on getting older, you master the art of yoga and all the skilled and prominent masters of yoga are very old aged people who have got all the control over these techniques and they are now teaching these techniques to their ancestors. Stamina increases with practice and people who have been practicing these techniques from young ages can become master of these arts in their older age.

Better Breathing And Body Awareness

When you keep on practicing yoga for longer periods of time then, you get a sense of awareness about your body and you know exactly what is going on inside your body. This helps you in identifying any faults and disorders very early in stage which helps to get rid of that disorder early.

With better breathing techniques, you feel comfortable and there are techniques in yoga which can enable you to attain relaxation in minutes. These techniques do not require any particular environment or timing and you can execute them even in your office chair to relax yourself.

Chapter 7:

Essentials for Doing Yoga at Home

Synopsis

There is some equipment which you need for the proper execution of yoga techniques and in this chapter I will tell you about that equipment.

- ☐ Yoga matt and its qualities
- ☐ Other miscellaneous yoga essentials

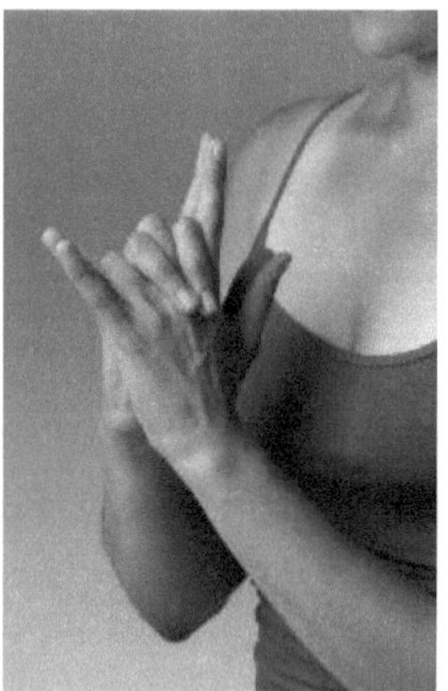

What You Need

If you have learned yoga and you want to practice now at home without bothering about going in classes then, you must have some essentials at home which will help you in executing your yoga techniques more effectively and more properly.

Yoga Matt and Its Qualities

Matt is the first essential thing which you must have in home and there are certain qualities of good quality yoga matt. First of all it should be very comfortable and smooth.

Thickness of matt also increases the comfort level but it will also increase the cost of matt. You can go with a medium thick matt for proper and healthy yoga practice.

You also should think about the cleaning method of your matt because if you are involved in hot yoga exercises then, matt will definitely get wet and will need to be washed. So look for a matt which you can wash in your washing machine easily.

Other Miscellaneous Yoga Essentials

Other than yoga matt, you should also carry a yoga bag and this is important because I have seen people who practice yoga that they do not care about their matt and towel and other things but you should have a proper bag which can hold all of your yoga items properly because discipline is first step of yoga and if you are not disciplined even in execution of yoga then, how can you expect any discipline in your life through yoga.

Some people will think that these essentials will cost them lots of money but believe it or not but all of the above items will not cost you more than $150. This is not a bog price to pay for proper execution of yoga in comfort of your house. So buy these accessories and exercise yoga at your home effectively.

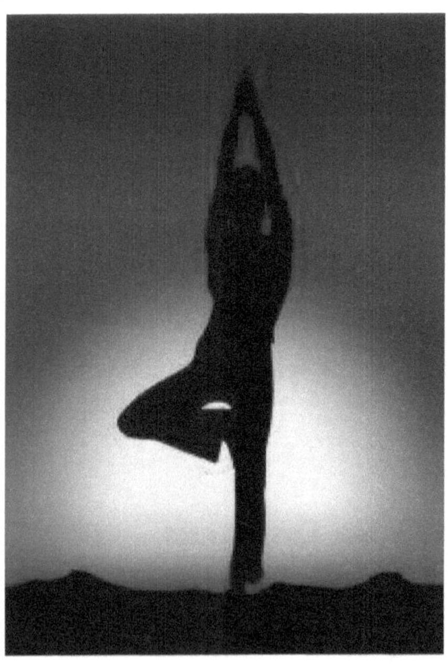

Wrapping up

In the above EBook, I have tried to tell you all about yoga practice and I am 100 percent sure that if you have read the whole book then, you will have started yoga at your own.

This is also necessary for your health and better than most of the ordinary and difficult exercise plans as it is cheapest exercise plan which you can adopt but once you decide to adopt it then, never leave your intention in half way and complete the whole process.

Once you start enjoying yoga then, everything will start to make sense because in start you will feel very awkward in bending your body and twisting your back but once you start getting the advantage and relaxation then, it will get better.

If you have been looking for inner peace and harmony for thoughts to achieve some serious goals in your life then, yoga can provide you with that kind of peace and liberty of thoughts.